The Chair to Your Successful Hair Journey

CHRISSY D. CARTER

THE CHAIR TO YOUR SUCCESSFUL HAIR JOURNEY

Please direct all copyright inquiries to:
B.O.Y. Publications, Inc.
c/o Author Copyrights
P.O. Box 262
Lowell, NC 28098
betonyourselfent.com

Paperback ISBN: 978-1-955605-63-2

Cover and Interior Design: B.O.Y. Enterprises, Inc.

Printed in the United States.

Dedication

I want to dedicate this book to my Lord and Savior Jesus Christ the very One Who inspired me to write this quick guide. To my beloved deceased grandmother, Annie Bell Hicklen, who help to open the door to my hair journey. I'm so very grateful for my loving husband and all our children, and my supportive mother. Lastly, I thank God for every client that I was graced to serve and the joy they brought to my life while operating behind the chair.

You Are Worthy

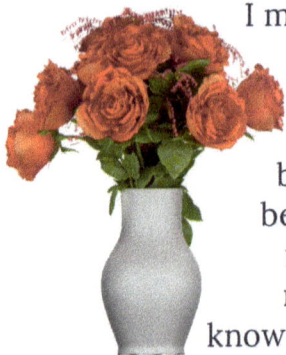

I must start out by saying something you may not hear often, but you are really worth it!! These roses..., well they are for you because, to me, you are absolutely beautiful! Being in the hair industry for almost 30 years I have seen so many beautiful women who didn't know they were beautiful because they didn't feel beautiful. Too often, we as women walk around not knowing our true value but today you must know, your worth is at an all-time high! It is for this reason alone, I decided to write this short "hair guidebook" just for you and your hair. Why Because not only are you worth it but your hair is worth it!

When I was in the hair industry I made sure I complimented my clients often. It was my reasonable service to empower them with my words, personal training on how to maintain the hair, product knowledge and them leaving the salon looking and feeling fabulous. So the fact that I'm no longer behind a chair, my assignment is to be an advocate for you, the client... empowering you with tools that will act as a "quick reference cheat sheet" that lands you in the right seat.

God put this guidebook in my heart some years ago and now I'm able to give something I believe will be valuable to you, the client. The reason I call this your cheat sheet is because my heart's desire is to cut out some leg work by getting the information directly to you. By the way, my name is Chrissy D Carter, I'm a native of Charlotte NC and I simply want you to win on this very important journey. So let's jump in and get you informed.

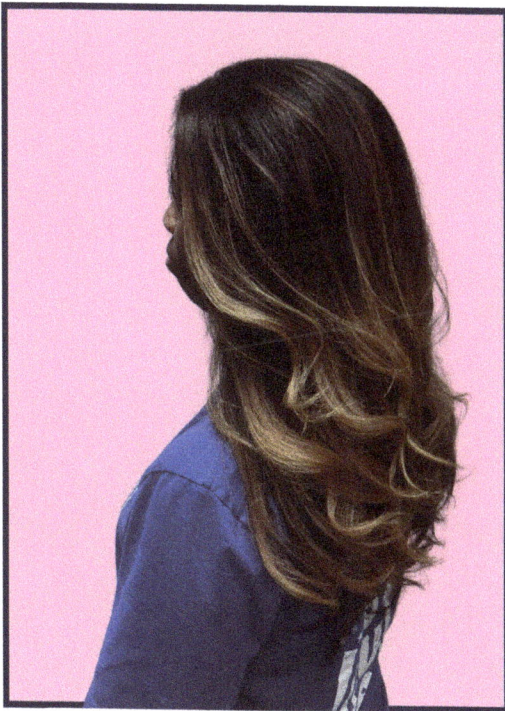

The Interview

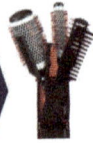

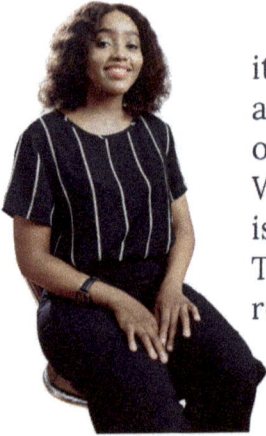

This is the make it or break it stage of your hair journey and I'm so grateful to be a part of something this monumental. Why...because not every chair is equipped to handle your hair. The key thing you must remember is, my hair is worth it and that it requires the best possible attention. Please remember this... "your hair will be the investment you make." The research, money, time, and love must come from you first and you will reap a good harvest!!

When it's consultation time, remember this is not just for the stylist to see if he or she can meet your needs, but this is also the hour for you to be in interview mode. Yes, you should be conducting your interview with this potential stylist. I don't know how many times in the past I have asked my clients important questions like, "What type of relaxer and what strength was used on your hair?

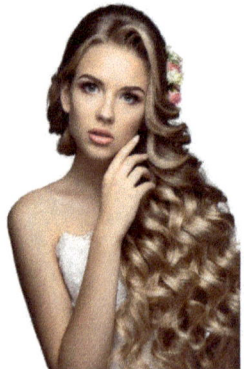

What type of products did the last stylist use?" Sadly, most of the time they didn't know. It's so important for you to be informed because these details have a great impact on the condition of your hair. It also gives your new stylist the history he or she needs to better service you to get your hair to its optimum healthy condition.

So it's important to ask questions. What type of products do you use? What strength relaxer would you use or recommend for my hair? How often should I get deep conditioners? What is your scheduling system like? Is there a wait time or will I be able to be seated in your chair at my scheduled time? This is not to be difficult but you do want to know if this relationship is going to cost you more than you can give. Your time is valuable and you need to know what type of environment you will be experiencing. Is this going to be the atmosphere that you can shake off the day and be in relax mode or is it full of gossip and chaotic?

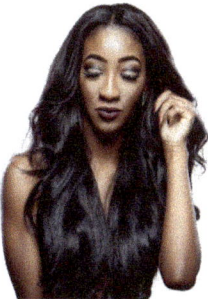

These things are important and only you know where your flexibility is and please make sure you are prayerful about areas of compromise.

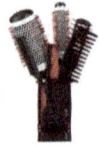

The Interview

Starting out, you must be the one stating what you are looking for in a "Healthy Hair Master Stylist" but the key here is knowing what to look for. That's where I come in...endowing you with knowledge and giving you some tools that will assist you on this journey.

Making sure you have the right fit is essential, therefore don't make the mistake of sitting in the chair of someone who is a master cut stylist but you want to grow your hair. This can be very conflicting and will at times lead to disappointment. Make sure you seek out, and I would advise you putting prayer on it, someone that concentrates on growing the hair. The majority of my clients came through prayer and for that reason alone we both reaped the benefits. I believe there should be a place of joy that comes from this relationship...just my personal stance.

I believe that when you do anything in love and joy, you will reap the harvest of healthy strong hair and I also believe that when there is stress, frustration, and dread...well the results will speak for themselves. Make sure this stylist loves what they do and it's not only about the money. That's a different topic for a different guidebook...lol. But make sure these areas are carefully regarded.

Key Things to Look For

OPEN AND INFORMATIVE: One of the things that set me apart as a "Healthy Master Stylist" is that I love teaching and educating my clients, so I walked them through the process and shared product knowledge. This is very important because it says your stylist desires to empower you and not handicap you by making you completely dependent on them. This has been proven to be very profitable for both parties and not only that but it builds a true bond. One of the things I believe, is that the right stylist wants you to be great even when they are not always accessible and that comes with them having a vision for your hair that's greater than their chair.

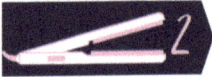

ORDER AND INFORMATION CARDS: This says everything about the character and integrity of the stylist. When there is order and things are not chaotic and unclean, this is a big plus because whatever you see...that's what you will get in return. You don't want to be just another number waiting to be seen but not seen. Remember you are worth this spa beauty treatment and that's exactly what your experience should be a spa treatment. That means your environment should take you away from all the hustle and bustle of it all and when you get to your appointment there should not be 1-2 hours of waiting with a wet head. This is a bad practice that's seen in too many salons where they have overbooked clients and the way to ensure the client doesn't leave is the "set you up to wait, shampoo method" but this is a poor representation of time stewardship.

There should also be records of your services to ensure proper tracking of chemicals, Keratin treatments and services in general. This speaks volumes because it says the stylist wants to administer the correct service and they want to create a visible timeline for your hair journey.

Key Things To Look For

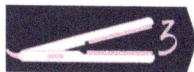

HIGH-END PRODUCTS: Simply put, because your hair is worth it, a great stylist will use the best! When I moved into my own salon, that was one of the first things the Lord spoke to me and that was to use the best hair products! It's what you put in that's going to determine your "breakthrough or your break-off!" Not only is using the good stuff important but it's a reasonable expectation for you as a paying client to know what's being used on your hair is top-notch. I had been in the industry going on 30 years and I have seen everything from a stylist burning off a customer's hair and putting it in their pocket to having a client request a certain relaxer and the stylist go to the back and put a different type of relaxer in a chemical bowl, thus deceiving the client. So it's important for you to know, see, and ask questions.

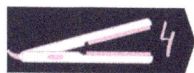

AN EVER-GROWING STYLIST: The right stylist is not satisfied with barely getting by, they pursue mastery skills! When it is their passion, there is fruit, evidence, or proof, and that's what you should look for. As they grow, so do you and your hair! An ever-growing stylist needs to be in the know about the latest techniques, services, and products, as well as what's good, and what's not.

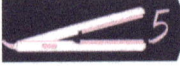

TIME IN PRAYER: This will always bring forth a harvest of peace and joy on your hair journey. When you are looking for optimum results there is work for you to do as well. My sole purpose for writing this quick reference hair guidebook is so you will be on the winning side when it comes to your hair. The picture you are viewing on the right is a client whose hair was transformed by my God-given knowledge of hair, using the right products, and her consistency in-home care and visits to my chair. You should always see visible progress!

Healthy Hair Journey

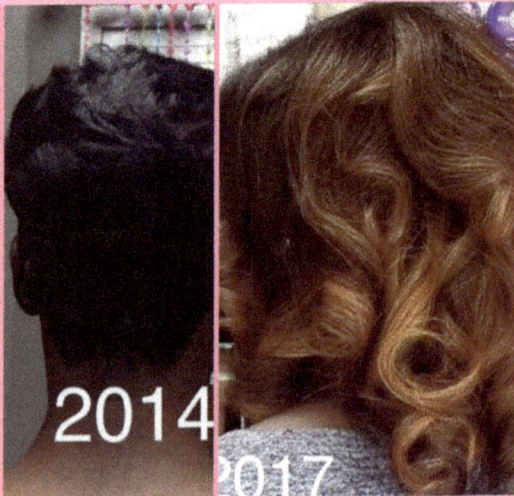

2014

2017

Bonus Tips

• Do your research and have a solid direction for your hair (put prayer on it). Sometimes you may need help getting there but at least know your objective (grow, cut or simply trying something different).

• Declutter and rid yourself of all the disappointments and know that no two stylist operate the same. If you have properly interviewed and researched your new stylist, their work should speak volumes. So trust the journey 😇

• Please, please purge your cabinets of old stale dated products and even check with your stylist to see if any of those products will work for your portion of maintenance. You don't want to be a product junky...it brings costly frustration that you don't need.

• Please, please be as dedicated to your hair journey as your stylist. When you receive the vision from your stylist let them know you are fully invested by your actions.

Bonus Tips Continued

• Stay hydrated with water, take vitamins (Biotin, vitamin E, B12), and make sure you check with your physician.

• Stimulation of the scalp for blood flow because this promotes growth. Some stylists disagree, but I'm the first partaker of this practice and it works.

• Always brush and comb your hair starting from the ends to the root using gentle strokes.

• Lastly, Speak life over your hair! Pray over your hair and watch God make the increase!

Customer Reviews

THE CHAIR TO YOUR SUCCESSFUL HAIR JOURNEY begins with a divinely appointed stylist. Therefore we must be careful of whom we trust with our crown. This divinely appointed stylist not only transforms you outwardly but inwardly as well. This occurs as he/she consults with the Father about your journey for your heavenly crown while assessing the condition of your natural crown. The impartation occurs during and in between appointments. THIS is what I experienced with MY divinely appointed stylist sent straight from heaven - Prophetess Chrissy Carter.

-BRENDA PIERCE

"**Transformative expertise paired with genuine care** - my journey from a closely shaved back to flourishing, long hair was guided by a remarkable hair stylist. Before a single tool touched my hair, Ms. Chrissy delved into conversations about my existing routine, water intake and product use. Our discussions extended beyond style, centering on healthy hair. With each thoughtful step, she sculpted a path for my hair's evolution, resulting in strands that reflect not just beauty but vitality. I am forever grateful for a stylist who listens, understands and empowers hair to thrive."

-THEANDRA THOMPSON

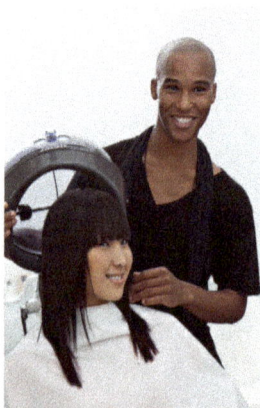

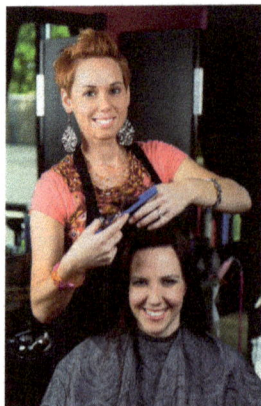

My Charlotte, NC Hair Journey

As a recent transplant to Charlotte for work, I had researched the neighborhood I wanted to live in before my work relocation; however, I did not research, via referral or word of mouth, where I could get my hair done. Transient life is not new for me as I had lived in several other locations throughout the United States and started my search to find a stylist in Charlotte as I've always done, by googling JC Penny Hair Salon near me.

Surprisingly, I've had decent outcomes with visiting a corporate entity that had staff on-hand who specialized in styling ethnic hair. Although my stylist at Carolina Place Mall was fairly decent, the energy exchange with the stylist was discordant and my hair, a living breathing organism on its own, was not that responsive to her either. So, I knew had to venture out to find some referrals; asking around, stopping into different salons and vetting their ethnic hair care experience. While looking for a stylist, I had begun to neglect my hair as I lost confidence in styling it myself. I wanted to change how I styled my hair with more healthy practices since the haircare world had changed dramatically since my days of using Climatress and Nexus products.

One Saturday, in a feat of desperation (my hair was on the verge of a cardiac arrest) I ran into every salon I could find within a mile radius of where I lived in the Arboretum neighborhood of Charlotte and found myself in Solas Salons. The African American woman at the front of Salon was able to get me in right away. This was my first indication that the something was a bit off. In demand stylists can never see you the minute you walk in. But I was desperate, so I went forward with sitting in her chair, with no expectations. While sitting in her chair, there was a flurry of traffic asking my stylist where they could find, Bold Hair (Prophetess Chrissy's Salon). I knew, right then, I had to find Bold Hair for myself. I asked my stylist who is this person these ladies are asking about. She didn't know but assumed, "she must be using Groupons." As soon as she finished, I made a beeline down the hall to find Bold Hair.

Prophetess Chrissy told me she had no availability and that I needed to make an appointment, which was music to my ears. I scheduled the first available appointment she had. She knew exactly how to style my soft, baby-fine hair. I didn't have to go home and "fix it" after having it styled. That was it for me. I began my every two weeks journey to her chair that day!

She took an inventory of my hair's current condition and completed a survey of how I had previously styled my hair; products used and how often, chemical services, etc. on a client worksheet. Any time a new process was introduced to my hair, she pulled out my client worksheet and updated it. Who does that?

When I left Charlotte, in 2019, my hair was the longest and healthiest it had been in my entire adult life. We take small things like a stylist for granted and we shouldn't. They should be vetted the same way we treat any other matters of significance. This encounter with a stylist who presumably lured in clients with Groupons, which was not the case, actually led to another world of fellowship and Spiritual renewal. It was more than my hair that grew while under her care. Today, our relationship is far beyond a client/ customer exchange and I'm forever grateful that my footsteps were ordered to "Bold Hair".

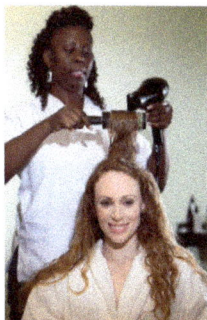

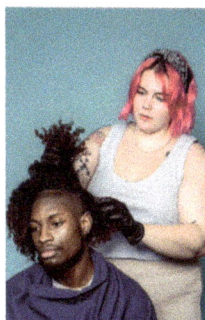